When The Body Speaks

Understanding Cleansing, Gut Health, and Individual Healing

Dr. Elena Rybak, PhD

Living Healthy Institute

This book is for educational purposes only and is not intended as a substitute for medical advice.

Printed in the United States of America

MEDICAL & EDUCATIONAL DISCLAIMER

This book is intended for educational and informational purposes only.

The content presented is not a substitute for professional medical advice, diagnosis, or treatment. The author is not a medical doctor, and the information contained herein should not be used to diagnose, treat, cure, or prevent any disease.

Always consult your physician or qualified healthcare provider before beginning any new dietary, nutritional, detoxification, fasting, or lifestyle program, especially if you are pregnant, nursing, taking medications, or have any medical condition.

The author and publisher assume no responsibility for any adverse effects resulting from the use or application of the information contained in this book.

Healing is individual, and what is appropriate for one person may not be appropriate for another.

Table of Contents

Table of Contents 1

Introduction 2

Chapter 1: The Digestive System — A System Under Pressure 6

Chapter 2: The Small Intestine — Where the Body Decides 9

Chapter 3: The Colon — Completion, Elimination, and Integrity 17

Chapter 4: Parasites — Hidden Burden, Subtle Signals.....23

Chapter 5: The Liver — Filtration, Flow, and Why It Must Be Seen First 31

Chapter 6: The Gallbladder — Storage, Release, and Preservation 39

Chapter 7: The Pancreas — Balance, Blood Sugar, and Burnout 47

Chapter 8: The Kidneys — Filtration, Balance, and Cleansing 55

Chapter 9: The Lymphatic System — Flow, Immunity, and Congestion 66

Chapter 10: Hormones — Thyroid, Adrenals, and Sex Hormones..73

Chapter 11: The Nervous System 80

Chapter 12: Diet and Nutrition — Simplicity, Purity, and Intelligent Nourishment 87

CONCLUSION...115

ABOUT THE AUTHOR..117

Introduction

When the Body Speaks

Healing does not begin with a diagnosis.
It begins with listening.

In my work, I have come to understand the body as an intelligent system — constantly processing, adapting, and communicating. Symptoms are not random events. They are signals that something within the system is under strain.

When people talk about "gut health," they often mean digestion alone. But in practice, the gut represents something broader. It is a central processing center where the body interprets what it takes in — physically, emotionally, and environmentally.

Food, stress, thoughts, emotions, and constant stimulation all enter the body through this system. When the load exceeds the body's ability to process, it does what it is designed to do: it stores, adapts, and compensates.

Symptoms arise not because the body is failing, but because it is trying to manage too much.

The Burden of Modern Life

The human body was not designed for the level of input we now experience daily.

Processed foods, chemical exposure, environmental pollution, emotional stress, and constant media consumption place an ongoing demand on the body's internal systems. There is little time to pause, reset, or fully process what is taken in.

Over time, this creates internal congestion — a buildup that is not only physical, but also emotional and energetic.

The early signs are often subtle:

- Reduced energy

- Digestive discomfort

- Mental fog

- Emotional reactivity

- A sense of imbalance

These are not failures. They are messages.

Internal Pollution Goes Beyond Toxins

Internal pollution is often thought of as chemical or environmental exposure. But the body also carries unprocessed stress, unresolved emotional experiences, and the energetic strain of constant stimulation.

The body does not distinguish between physical and emotional input. What is not processed is held — and what is held eventually affects function.

This book is not about blaming modern life or creating fear. It is about understanding how the body responds to sustained pressure — and why so many people feel depleted, inflamed, or disconnected despite doing their best to live well.

Understanding Comes Before Change

Healing is not something that can be forced. It begins with understanding what the body has been carrying.

This book is meant to inform, not instruct. It offers insight into how the body processes life, why symptoms develop, and why healing must always be individualized.

We begin with the digestive system — not because it is trendy, but because it is foundational.

The body is always speaking.
Learning to listen changes everything.

Chapter 1: The Digestive System — A System Under Pressure

The digestive system is responsible for one of the most essential tasks in the body: turning what we consume into nourishment and eliminating what does not belong.

This process requires coordination, timing, and nervous system support. When digestion functions well, it operates quietly in the background. When it does not, the effects can be felt throughout the entire body.

A System, Not a Single Organ

Digestion is not the job of one organ. It is a sequence involving multiple structures working together.

Each part has a specific role:

- The **stomach** prepares food for absorption

- The **small intestine** absorbs nutrients

- The **liver and gallbladder** assist in fat processing and filtration

- The **pancreas** supplies digestive enzymes

- The **colon** eliminates waste

When this sequence is disrupted, efficiency declines and the system compensates.

The Nervous System Sets the Tone

Digestion depends on the nervous system.

When the body feels safe and regulated, digestion is supported. When the body is under stress, digestion slows. Blood flow shifts, enzyme production decreases, and movement through the digestive tract changes.

This is why digestive symptoms often appear during periods of emotional or mental strain — even when diet remains unchanged.

In modern life, many people live in a constant state of low-level stress. Over time, this alone can compromise digestion.

Compensation Creates Strain

When digestion becomes inefficient, the body adapts.

One organ works harder to make up for another. Waste remains in the system longer than intended. Absorption becomes less effective.

Over time, this compensation creates physical strain within the digestive system and contributes to broader patterns of imbalance involving energy, immunity, and inflammation.

Digestive symptoms rarely exist alone.

Why Isolated Approaches Often Fail

Because digestion functions as a system, addressing one symptom or one organ often brings only temporary relief.

Supporting digestion requires understanding how the system works together and why it has become strained in the first place.

This understanding prepares us to look more closely at the organ that plays the most decisive role in nourishment and discernment.

Chapter 2: The Small Intestine — Where the Body Decides

The small intestine is where nourishment truly occurs.

Health is not determined by how much food is consumed, but by how well nutrients are absorbed. The small intestine is responsible for this task, making it one of the most critical organs in the body.

When absorption is impaired, the body may receive food but remain undernourished.

How It Works

- **Digestion & Nutrient Absorption:** The small intestine receives partially digested food from the stomach. Pancreatic enzymes and bile mix with the chyme to break down proteins, fats, and carbohydrates.

- **Villi & Microvilli:** The inner surface of the small intestine is covered in tiny finger-like projections called villi, which increase the surface area for absorption. Microvilli on each villus further maximize contact with nutrients, ensuring vitamins, minerals, amino acids, and fatty acids are absorbed efficiently into the bloodstream.

- **Transport to Organs:** Nutrients absorbed here are distributed to organs and tissues according to need. This system ensures each organ receives the exact nutrients required for energy, repair, and optimal function.

When Function Is Compromised

- **Clogged Villi:** Mucus, residues, or toxins can coat the villi, preventing proper absorption. Nutrients are lost, energy declines, and organs may become deficient in essential compounds.

- **Leaky Gut:** When the intestinal lining is damaged, gaps form between cells. These gaps allow undigested food particles, toxins, and microbes to enter the bloodstream, triggering inflammation, immune reactions, and systemic stress. Chronic leaky gut can lead to fatigue, skin issues, food sensitivities, and autoimmune problems.

- **Immune and Emotional Consequences:** Because 70% of immune cells reside in the gut, compromised small intestine function weakens immunity. Emotional memory stored in this organ may intensify, manifesting as anxiety, mood swings, or unexplained emotional release during cleansing procedures.

Absorption Is the Foundation of Health

The lining of the small intestine is designed to maximize absorption. Through this surface, nutrients enter the bloodstream and are delivered to every cell.

When this process is compromised, deficiencies can develop even with a balanced diet. Fatigue, weakness, and imbalance often follow — not because of lack of effort, but because nourishment is not reaching where it is needed.

A Center of Discernment

In traditional Chinese medicine, the small intestine is understood as a primary center of discernment — responsible for separating what is useful from what is not.

In this framework, the brain processes information, while the body processes experience.

Emotional memory is not stored as thoughts alone. It is carried in the body, particularly within the organs.

Emotional Load and Physical Function

The small intestine is highly sensitive to sustained emotional and mental pressure.

Chronic stress, internal tension, and constant stimulation place ongoing demand on this organ. Over time, this strain can interfere with both physical absorption and emotional processing.

Internal congestion often begins quietly — long before physical symptoms appear.

What I Have Observed in Practice

During guided small intestine work in my practice, physical release is sometimes accompanied by emotional release.

Some individuals begin to cry or experience a sudden outpouring of emotion without a clear reason or memory attached. There are often no words, no explanations — and none are needed.

In these moments, I do not encourage analysis. I suggest allowing the body to do what it is ready to do.

I have witnessed strong, grounded individuals soften completely — not from weakness, but from release. These experiences are natural, unforced, and deeply settling.

The Body's Quiet Intelligence

The body releases what it is prepared to release.

Healing does not always arrive with understanding or language. Sometimes it arrives as relief, lightness, or calm — without explanation.

The small intestine is not only an organ of digestion. It is a place of decision, integration, and release.

Understanding its role helps explain why healing so often begins here — and why guidance, readiness, and respect for the body matter.

Small Intestine — Absorption, Assimilation, and Internal Clarity

The small intestine determines what the body keeps and what it cannot use.

When it is congested, inflamed, or burdened, even the best food becomes waste.

These foods are designed to:

- reduce mucus
- support villi function
- calm irritation
- improve nutrient uptake
- support leaky-gut repair

Healing Carrot–Celery Juice

Purpose:
Anti-parasitic, anti-fungal, mucus-dissolving, villi-supportive

Ingredients:
- *5–6 carrots*
- *2–3 celery stalks*

How to use:
Juice fresh. Drink on empty stomach only.

Support:

This combination cleans the intestinal lining, improves bile interaction, and enhances absorption efficiency.

Soothing Intestinal Porridge

Purpose:

Repair, calm, rebuild, and nourish intestinal lining

Ingredients:

- *½ cup cooked buckwheat or quinoa*
- *Steamed zucchini or pumpkin*
- *A drizzle of olive oil*
- *Pinch of sea salt*

Why it helps:

Warm, soft, mineral-rich, non-irritating.

Ideal during healing phases and digestive weakness.

Green Absorption Juice

Purpose:

Amino acids for blood, enzyme support, inflammation reduction

Ingredients:

- *Cucumber*
- *Celery*
- *Spinach or parsley*
- *Lemon*

Use:

Morning or mid-day on empty stomach.

Chapter 3: The Colon — Completion, Elimination, and Integrity

If the small intestine absorbs and decides what the body keeps, the colon completes the process. It is the final stage of the digestive system, responsible for eliminating what the body no longer needs: waste, toxins, and byproducts of metabolism.

The colon is often overlooked because it works quietly in the background. Yet when it is congested or sluggish, the effects are felt throughout the entire body, physically, emotionally, and energetically.

The Colon: The Body's Sewer

The colon functions as the body's primary sewer. Its role is to remove waste efficiently and prevent toxins from lingering. This is crucial because the blood supply from the colon travels through the rest of the body. Toxins that remain in the colon do not stay there; they can enter the bloodstream and be transported to other organs, affecting the liver, kidneys, heart, and brain.

A clogged colon also expands, placing pressure on surrounding organs, reducing circulation, and compromising blood flow. Over time, this contributes to fatigue, organ strain, and impaired detoxification. For this reason, regular support of the colon is not optional, it is essential for maintaining systemic health and supporting the body's natural cleansing processes.

The Colon's Role in Health

The colon is far more than a simple "exit tube." It absorbs water and electrolytes, consolidates waste for elimination, maintains a healthy balance of gut flora, and supports immune function through the gut-immune connection. When the colon functions efficiently, elimination is smooth, energy is higher, and the body's detoxification pathways remain supported.

When the Colon Becomes Congested

Colon function can be slowed by many common lifestyle factors, including low fiber or highly processed diets, dehydration, sedentary habits, chronic stress and emotional tension, and overload from inefficiency in the liver and small intestine.

The consequences of this congestion often include constipation or irregular elimination, bloating and abdominal discomfort, fatigue, toxin reabsorption when waste remains too long in the body, and an increased inflammatory burden. Even minor stagnation can ripple through the system, affecting digestion, mood, and overall vitality.

The Colon and Emotional Health

In traditional and holistic systems, the colon is associated with the ability to let go, both physically and emotionally. When elimination is impaired, people frequently report a sense of heaviness, emotional stagnation, and difficulty releasing old patterns or stress. Supporting the colon encourages not only physical release, but also the restoration of natural rhythm and internal flow.

Supporting the Colon Naturally

Healthy colon function depends on more than laxatives or occasional detoxes. It requires adequate hydration, fiber-rich foods such as fruits, vegetables, and whole grains, regular movement to stimulate intestinal motility, support of the microbiome through fermented foods, prebiotics, and probiotics, and effective stress management. Chronic tension directly slows peristalsis and impairs elimination.

When these factors are addressed, the colon supports the entire digestive system, complementing nutrient absorption in the small intestine and detoxification in the liver and gallbladder.

What I Have Observed in Practice

Even small improvements in colon function often lead to meaningful changes in overall well-being. Energy increases, bloating and discomfort decrease, skin clarity improves, sleep quality improves, and emotional balance becomes more stable. A well-functioning colon sets the stage for deeper healing throughout the body by ensuring that nutrients are properly utilized and toxins are removed rather than recycled.

The Colon as a Final Checkpoint

The colon is the body's final checkpoint. It is the last opportunity to eliminate what is no longer needed so that the upstream systems, the liver, gallbladder, pancreas, and small intestine, can function without interference.

Supporting colon health is not about quick fixes. It is about consistency, gentle care, and respect for the body's natural rhythms.

Intestinal Repair Soup

Purpose:

Reduce irritation, support mucosa, improve transit

Ingredients:
* *Zucchini*
* *Celery*

- *Carrot*

- *Onion*

- *Parsley*

- *Olive oil*

Simmer gently, blend if needed.

Simple Digestive Plate

Purpose:

Prevent overload, support clean digestion

Plate idea:

- *Steamed vegetables*
- *Small portion of whole grain (quinoa, buckwheat)*
- *Olive oil & herbs*

Chapter 4: Parasites — Hidden Burden, Subtle Signals

Parasites are often assumed to be rare or exotic — something contracted only through travel or extreme exposure. In reality, they are far more common than most people realize. It is estimated that there are nearly two hundred different types of parasites capable of living in the human body, affecting not only the digestive tract but also tissues, organs, and systemic function.

Because of this diversity, it is practically impossible to test for every parasite species. Many people carry low-level parasitic or microbial burdens without ever receiving a clear diagnosis, yet still experience chronic symptoms that point to deeper imbalance.

A Silent Presence

Parasites do not always announce themselves dramatically. Many exist quietly, drawing resources, irritating tissues, and interfering with normal digestive and immune processes. A single female roundworm can lay hundreds of thousands of eggs over short periods of time, allowing populations to expand rapidly once conditions are favorable.

While cooking temperatures may destroy live worms, parasite eggs are far more resilient and often survive common food preparation. When consumed, they may remain dormant for years — sometimes decades — waiting for the right internal conditions to hatch.

Immune Stress and Activation

The immune system plays a crucial role in keeping parasitic activity in check. As long as immune function remains strong and the internal environment is balanced, many organisms remain inactive.

However, when immunity becomes compromised — through chronic stress, emotional overload, illness, exhaustion, or antibiotic use — dormant organisms may activate. At that point, infestation occurs not necessarily because of new exposure, but because the internal terrain has changed.

This explains why symptoms often appear suddenly and without an obvious external cause.

Antibiotics and Microbial Imbalance

Antibiotics, while sometimes necessary, do not discriminate between harmful and beneficial organisms. Their use disrupts protective intestinal flora and weakens one of the body's most important defense systems.

In this altered environment, parasites, yeast, and pathogenic bacteria gain opportunity to proliferate. Balance does not automatically restore itself once medication is stopped. The digestive ecosystem often requires intentional rebuilding.

How Parasites Enter the Body

Parasites are present throughout the environment and enter the body through multiple pathways:

• Food that is improperly washed, handled, or undercooked.

• Water that is contaminated or insufficiently purified.

• Airborne particles and dust.

• Soil and insect contact.

• Animals and household pets.

• Close personal contact and shared surfaces.

• Travel and environmental exposure.

Modern hygiene does not eliminate these pathways. It only reduces their visibility.

Where Parasites Thrive

Approximately ninety percent of parasites affecting humans reside in the gastrointestinal tract, particularly the small intestine, where nutrients are abundant and easily accessible.

Others may inhabit nearly any tissue, including the liver, lungs, brain, blood, muscles, joints, skin, and vascular system.

They favor environments that are toxic, inflamed, nutritionally imbalanced, and immunologically weakened.

How Parasites Harm the Body

Parasites compromise health in several fundamental ways:

• They release metabolic waste and toxins into the blood, lymph, and digestive tract.

• They physically damage tissues and intestinal lining.

- They trigger inflammatory and allergic reactions, especially during die-off phases.

- They consume vitamins, minerals, enzymes, hormones, and blood.

- They weaken immune function and increase disease susceptibility.

The result may appear as fatigue, digestive disturbance, skin disorders, allergies, mood imbalance, nutrient deficiencies, cravings, and chronic inflammatory conditions.

Why Testing Is Often Inconclusive

Parasites exist in cycles and stages that are difficult to capture through conventional testing. They may hide within tissues, remain dormant, or shed intermittently.

For this reason, absence of detection does not equate to absence of burden. Clinical observation, symptom patterns, digestive function, immune resilience, and elimination capacity often provide more meaningful insight than laboratory results alone.

A Thoughtful and Prepared Approach

Addressing parasites without proper preparation can overwhelm the body. When digestion, bile flow, liver function, lymphatic drainage, and elimination pathways are compromised, aggressive interventions may create more harm than benefit.

A guided and sequential approach allows the body to:

• Strengthen digestion

• Support detoxification pathways

• Restore microbial balance

• Reduce inflammatory load

When addressed at the right time and in the right context, parasite support becomes restorative rather than disruptive.

What I Have Observed in Practice

I have repeatedly seen individuals who suffered for years with vague digestive issues, immune instability, fatigue, and unexplained symptoms experience meaningful improvement once parasitic burden was addressed — but only after foundational systems were supported. Parasites are rarely the sole cause. They are part of a larger pattern of internal overload.

Not an Enemy — A Signal

Parasites are not something to fear. They are a signal that the body has been under strain and requires support.

When approached with understanding and respect for the body's intelligence, their presence becomes a doorway into deeper healing rather than a source of alarm.

DETOX PARASITES GENTLY ON DAILY BASIS HELPFUL TIPS:

Consume onions in your salads, garlic raw and cooked. Add garlic powder to every soup or dish you cook.

Ginger in every way is great.

Cranberries have powerful anti parasitic qualities.

Pumpkin seeds are great for their nutrition and amount of zinc but they are also to attract and then remove intestinal parasites. Eating a handful of pumpkin seeds daily on empty stomach is beneficial.

You can also make pumpkin seed milk:

2 table spoons of seeds.

2 cups of water.

Bland until smooth.

Drink as is or run through s trainer for a smoother feel. Can add some honey for sweetness.

Chapter 5: The Liver — Filtration, Flow, and Why It Must Be Seen First

If the small intestine decides what the body keeps, the liver determines how the body processes what it cannot avoid, and how well the body releases what it no longer needs.

The liver is one of the most resilient and capable organs in the human body. It is highly adaptive and uniquely designed to regenerate itself. Given the right environment, the liver has the capacity to rebuild its own tissue, a remarkable feature unmatched by most other organs.

But in our current conditions, the liver carries a burden far greater than what it evolved to manage.

What the Liver Actually Does

The liver performs dozens of essential functions simultaneously. It filters and cleanses the blood, processes chemicals, environmental exposures, and medications, assists in hormone regulation, regulates blood sugar, produces bile for fat digestion, and supports immune function.

Everything you eat, breathe, absorb through the skin, or experience emotionally eventually passes through this organ. Because the liver's responsibilities are so broad, its function affects nearly every system in the body, especially digestion, immunity, and nervous system balance.

Why Liver Overload Is So Common

In an ideal state, without constant exposure to processed foods, environmental toxins, medications, and chronic emotional stress, the liver would complete a natural regeneration cycle approximately every six months. This is not theoretical; it is part of its biological design.

Most people, however, never give the liver the opportunity to reset. Heavy meals late in the evening, chemically burdened foods, unresolved emotional stress, daily environmental exposure, and continuous stimulation prevent the liver from entering its restorative phase.

The liver is a night organ. Its deepest work occurs during rest, sleep, and repair cycles. When it is still digesting heavy food in the evening, it cannot shift into regeneration mode. Its energy remains focused on processing intake rather than clearing stored waste and toxins. This is one reason many people wake feeling tired, congested, or inflamed: the liver never had the space to repair.

Allergies as a Sign of Liver Pollution

Food sensitivities, seasonal allergies, and environmental reactions are not random events. When the liver is burdened with toxins, chemicals, and excess metabolic waste, it becomes less efficient at processing proteins, histamines, and inflammatory compounds.

This often presents as food sensitivities, hay fever, skin reactions, sinus congestion, and respiratory irritation. Because the immune system is closely tied to the liver's capacity to clear antigens, allergic responses increase when liver function is compromised. In practice, improving liver flow frequently leads to a significant reduction in allergy symptoms.

Liver Regeneration — Possible, But Blocked

The liver is designed to regenerate. Healthy organisms naturally allow this through periods of rest and reduced intake. Humans evolved with similar rhythms.

In modern life, however, heavy evening eating, chronic stress, fragmented sleep, and continuous emotional and environmental stimulation prevent the liver from entering this deeper restorative state. Instead of regeneration, the liver remains in a constant backlog.

The Consequences of Working Without Pause

When regeneration is blocked, the stress is distributed throughout the body. This often manifests as fatigue, hormonal imbalance, poor fat digestion, sluggish bile flow, constipation, emotional irritability, frequent allergies, immune sensitivity, brain fog, and reduced resilience. These symptoms are not isolated. They reflect the liver's inability to meet the cumulative load placed upon it.

Why a Proper Liver Cleanse Matters

Not all liver cleanses are equal. Many provide only temporary support through hydration or mild stimulation without addressing deeper congestion.

A true, guided liver cleanse supports the safe release of stored materials, encourages bile flow, maintains balanced detox pathways, and allows the liver to shift from constant processing into regenerative function.

In my experience, this is one of the most transformative steps in healing. Properly supported liver cleansing changes the function of the entire body. As liver flow improves, digestion becomes easier, energy increases, immunity stabilizes, mood sharpens, and the body's innate intelligence begins to reassert itself.

Support and Supervision Matter

Because the liver is central to all systems, supporting it requires respect for the individual body, correct timing and sequence, careful monitoring, and awareness of unique responses. This is not a one-size-fits-all approach.

Supervised cleansing is essential for both safety and lasting results.

The Liver as a Bridge

When liver function improves, digestive efficiency increases, emotional resilience deepens, sleep becomes more restorative, allergic tendencies decrease, hormones stabilize, and energy becomes steadier.

The liver is not only a filter. It is a bridge connecting digestion, elimination, immunity, metabolism, stress response, and emotional integration.

Supporting it intelligently is not optional. It is foundational.

Liver — Filtration, Flow, and Regeneration Support

The liver responds best to foods that are:
• light
• bitter
• mineral-rich

- fluid

- non-congesting

The goal is to thin bile, move stored waste, reduce inflammatory load, and allow regeneration.

Classic Liver Cleanse Juice

Purpose:

Bile stimulation, stone-softening, detox support

Ingredients:

- *3 carrots*

- *1 beet*

- *1 green apple*

- *Lemon*

How to use:

Drink twice daily on empty stomach during liver-support phases.

Bitter Green Juice

Purpose:

Stimulate liver enzymes, improve fat digestion, reduce congestion

Ingredients:

- *Celery*

- *Dandelion greens or arugula*
- *Cucumber*
- *Lemon*

Liver-Supportive Salad

Purpose:
Mineral replenishment, gentle detox

Base:
- *Mixed greens*
- *Beet slices*
- *Cucumber*
- *Olive oil & lemon*

Regeneration Drink

Purpose:
Mineralization & bile quality support

Ingredients:
- *Warm water*
- *Lemon*
- *Pinch Celtic salt*

Morning tonic.

Chapter 6: The Gallbladder — Storage, Release, and Preservation

The gallbladder is often overlooked, yet it plays a critical role in digestion, detoxification, and metabolic balance. Working in close partnership with the liver, it stores and concentrates bile, a substance essential for digesting fats and carrying waste out of the body.

Though small, its function influences digestion, blood sugar regulation, and long-term metabolic health. When the gallbladder becomes congested, the effects extend far beyond digestive discomfort.

The Gallbladder's Role in Digestion and Detoxification

Bile is produced by the liver, but it is the gallbladder that stores, concentrates, and releases it when needed.

Bile breaks down fats, allows absorption of fat-soluble nutrients, binds to toxins and waste, and supports efficient elimination. When bile quality declines or release becomes

impaired, digestion suffers and toxins remain in circulation
longer than intended.

How Gallbladder Stones Form

Gallbladder stones develop when toxins, excess cholesterol,
metabolic waste, and thickened bile accumulate over time.
As the liver becomes burdened, bile can lose its natural
fluidity.

When the gallbladder is unable to properly purify and
release this bile, material begins to settle and harden. Stone
formation is not sudden; it reflects long-term congestion and
reduced cleansing capacity.

In early stages, this process may go unnoticed. As stones
grow larger, symptoms can appear, including pain or
pressure under the right rib, digestive distress after fatty
meals, nausea, and sudden gallbladder "attacks." At this
stage, many people are told that removal of the gallbladder
is the only option.

Preservation Is Often Possible

In my practice, I have seen that with proper preparation and professional guidance, the gallbladder can often be preserved. I have worked with individuals diagnosed with large gallstones, including stones measuring approximately 5 to 10 cm in diameter based on ultrasound findings. Through a structured and supervised approach, these individuals were able to release stones gradually and safely, and follow-up imaging showed no remaining stones.

This process is not a quick fix. It requires the right preparatory phase, dietary changes to reduce bile thickness, juicing and herbal support, gradual reduction in stone size, and careful timing and supervision.

Attempting this without guidance can be ineffective or unsafe, but when done correctly, preserving this organ is often worth the commitment. The gallbladder is not expendable, it is functional.

When the Gallbladder Has Been Removed

When the gallbladder has already been removed, people are often told they can now "eat whatever they want," because pain is no longer present. While symptoms may disappear, the underlying workload does not.

Without a gallbladder, bile is no longer stored and released in a controlled manner. The digestive system adapts, and the pancreas often compensates by taking on additional digestive and metabolic demand.

Over time, this added burden commonly contributes to blood sugar instability, hypoglycemia, insulin resistance, and metabolic strain. These changes are not immediate, but they are patterns I have observed repeatedly.

Why Liver Support Becomes Even More Important

In the absence of a gallbladder, the liver's role becomes even more critical. Bile quality, detoxification efficiency, and metabolic regulation depend heavily on liver function.

Supporting the liver is no longer optional, it becomes essential.

In these cases, careful attention to clean, organic, and lean foods, appropriate meal timing, digestive support, juicing, and gentle, guided cleansing becomes increasingly important for long-term balance.

Preservation Over Removal

The gallbladder's role in digestion, detoxification, and metabolic flow is significant. When preservation is possible, it supports better fat digestion, reduces strain on the pancreas, improves toxin elimination, and strengthens metabolic resilience.

Healing is not about silencing symptoms. It is about restoring function.

The Gallbladder as a Turning Point

The gallbladder represents the body's ability to release, both physically and metabolically. When supported appropriately, many people experience improved digestion, greater energy stability, reduced inflammatory response, and increased resilience.

Understanding and respecting this organ changes how we approach healing.

Gallbladder — Storage, Release, and Stone Reduction Support

The gallbladder needs foods that:
- thin bile
- reduce stagnation
- soften congestion
- support rhythmic release

These recipes are designed to prepare the system, not force it.

Potato Water Preparation (Stone-Softening Protocol)

Indication: Diagnosed gallbladder stones

Preparation:
Wash thoroughly **2 lb potatoes (do not peel)**.
Cover with **3 quarts water**.

Boil until liquid is reduced by half.

Mash potatoes and leave overnight.

In the morning, strain and keep the liquid.

Use:

*Drink **4 oz before each meal***

*For **1–2 weeks prior to liver/gallbladder cleansing.***

Purpose:

Softens bile, reduces stone density, and prepares the gallbladder for safer release.

Bile-Flow Juice

Purpose:

Improve bile movement and fat digestion.

Ingredients:

- *Celery*
- *Cucumber*
- *Lemon*
- *Small piece of ginger*

Drink on empty stomach.

Light Digestive Soup

Purpose:

Reduce gallbladder workload.

Ingredients:

- *Zucchini*
- *Carrot*
- *Onion*
- *Parsley*

Warm, simple, and evening-friendly.

Gallbladder-Friendly Plate

Purpose:

Prevent bile thickening.

Plate idea:

- *Steamed vegetables*
- *Quinoa or buckwheat*
- *Olive oil & lemon*

Avoid heavy fats, fried foods, and late dinners during support phases.

Chapter 7: The Pancreas — Balance, Blood Sugar, and Burnout

The pancreas is a quiet organ that works constantly behind the scenes. It rarely demands attention — until it is overwhelmed.

Positioned between digestion and metabolism, the pancreas plays a central role in regulating blood sugar, producing digestive enzymes, and maintaining energy balance. When this organ is strained, the effects are widespread and often misunderstood.

Understanding the pancreas is essential to understanding fatigue, blood sugar instability, and metabolic burnout.

The Dual Role of the Pancreas

The pancreas has two primary responsibilities:

1. **Digestive support** — producing enzymes that help break down carbohydrates, fats, and proteins

2. **Blood sugar regulation** — releasing insulin and glucagon to maintain stable energy levels

These functions must remain finely balanced. When the pancreas is asked to compensate for other organ dysfunction, that balance is disrupted.

When the Pancreas Takes on Too Much

When bile flow is impaired or the gallbladder is absent, the pancreas often increases enzyme output to assist digestion.

At the same time, modern diets high in refined carbohydrates and irregular eating patterns force the pancreas to release insulin repeatedly throughout the day.

This combination places enormous stress on an organ that was never designed for constant output without rest.

Over time, this may contribute to:

- Blood sugar swings

- Hypoglycemia

- Insulin resistance

- Fatigue after meals

- Cravings and energy crashes

These symptoms are often treated in isolation, without addressing the underlying workload placed on the pancreas.

The Link Between Digestion and Blood Sugar

Digestion and blood sugar regulation are inseparable.

When food is poorly digested, nutrients enter the bloodstream unevenly. This creates spikes and crashes that force the pancreas to work harder to stabilize levels.

If the liver and gallbladder are congested, this imbalance intensifies. The pancreas becomes a compensatory organ — doing more work to keep the system functioning.

Burnout Happens Quietly

Pancreatic strain does not usually announce itself early.

It develops gradually, as the organ responds to years of:

- Dietary overload

- Irregular meal timing

- Liver and gallbladder congestion

- Chronic stress

By the time blood sugar issues are diagnosed, the pancreas has often been compensating for a long time.

This is why addressing blood sugar without addressing digestion and liver function often brings only partial relief.

What I Have Seen in Practice

In practice, I frequently see blood sugar imbalance improve only after liver and gallbladder function are supported.

When the pancreas no longer has to compensate for poor bile flow or impaired digestion, its workload decreases — and balance becomes possible again.

This is not about forcing insulin levels. It is about restoring proper sequence and support within the system.

Why Pancreatic Support Requires a Broader View

The pancreas does not function independently.

Supporting this organ requires:

- Reducing digestive strain

- Supporting liver filtration

- Improving bile flow

- Respecting timing and rest

Without these foundations, efforts focused solely on blood sugar often fall short.

The Pancreas as a Warning System

Pancreatic symptoms often signal that the body has been compensating for too long.

They are not the beginning of imbalance — they are a later message.

Listening at this stage can prevent deeper metabolic dysfunction and long-term consequences.

Preparing for Completion

With digestion, absorption, filtration, release, and metabolic regulation understood, the final step in the gut system is elimination.

Later in this book, we will return to the colon — not as an isolated organ, but as a reflection of how well the entire system has been supported.

The body does not rush healing.

It restores balance when pressure is reduced.

Pancreas — Enzyme Support & Blood Sugar Balance

The pancreas is stressed primarily by:

- excess sugar
- refined carbohydrates
- heavy animal proteins
- irregular eating
- chronic stimulation

Its healing requires simplicity, mineral balance, and steady glucose input.

Blood Sugar Stabilizing Green Juice

Purpose: *Reduce insulin spikes, nourish pancreatic tissue.*

Ingredients:

- *Cucumber*
- *Celery*
- *Spinach*
- *Lemon*

Enzyme Support Broth

Purpose: Reduce digestive demand on pancreas.

Ingredients:

- Zucchini
- Fennel
- Onion
- Parsley

Warm, light, restorative.

Pancreas-Friendly Breakfast Bowl

Purpose: Gentle glucose release.

Ingredients:

- Buckwheat
- Stewed apple (no sugar)
- Cinnamon

Metabolic Support Drink

Purpose: Improve insulin sensitivity.

Ingredients:

- Warm water

- *Apple cider vinegar*
- *Pinch Celtic salt*

Stabilizing Plate

Purpose: *Prevent glycemic overload.*

Plate idea:
- *Steamed vegetables*
- *Lentils or quinoa*
- *Olive oil*

Chapter 8: The Kidneys — Filtration, Balance, and Cleansing

The kidneys are vital organs that work quietly and constantly to keep the body balanced. They filter the blood, remove waste, regulate fluid levels, balance minerals, support hormone production, and maintain the delicate interplay between acidity and alkalinity in the body. Kidneys are not just filters — they are *essential regulators* of the internal environment.

Every day, kidneys process large volumes of blood, separating what the body needs from what it no longer requires. The waste that is filtered out becomes urine, and the "cleaned" blood continues circulating throughout the body. This filtration process is central to overall health — and when it becomes burdened, the effects ripple outward.

What the Kidneys Do

The kidneys perform multiple intertwined functions:

- **Filter and purify blood:** They remove toxins, metabolic waste, and excess substances.

- **Regulate fluid balance:** They determine how much fluid the body retains and how much is excreted.

- **Balance minerals and electrolytes:** These include sodium, potassium, calcium, and magnesium.

- **Support acid–alkaline balance:** This balance is crucial for metabolic and enzymatic processes.

- **Produce hormones:** They help regulate blood pressure and support red blood cell production.

These roles are continuous — the kidneys never stop working. As long as a person is alive, the kidneys are filtering, balancing, and regulating.

Why the Kidneys Become Overloaded

Just like the liver, the kidneys are designed to manage a certain level of physical and environmental stress. But modern life — with processed foods, chemical exposures, chronic dehydration, and emotional stress — places extraordinary demand on these organs.

When too much burdened material passes through the system, the kidneys struggle to keep up. For example, mineral deposits can accumulate within the kidneys, leading to stones. Salt, chemicals, acidic waste, and poor hydration make it more difficult for the kidneys to filter efficiently.

Over time, this overload can contribute to:

- Sluggish filtration

- Imbalanced fluids and minerals

- Lower back discomfort

- Increased pressure on the heart and cardiovascular system

- Higher metabolic stress

- Immune strain

When kidneys are overworked, wastes that should be eliminated linger in the body longer than intended, increasing toxic load and overall systemic stress.

Kidney Function Affects the Whole Body

The kidneys do more than remove waste. Because they regulate blood composition, fluid balance, and mineral levels, their function influences many systems, including:

- **Blood pressure regulation**

- **Bone health**

- **Hormonal balance**

- **Immune function**

- **Nervous system stability**

- **Sleep and energy cycles**

When the kidneys are sluggish, the body reacts. Toxins that should have been eliminated stay in circulation longer. The immune system works harder. Other organs — like the liver and heart — must compensate. This cascading impact is why kidney function plays such an influential role in overall wellness.

Cleansing the Kidneys — What It Entails

Cleansing the kidneys is not a trendy shortcut or a superficial ritual. It is a *supportive process* designed to reduce the accumulated burden that can overwhelm filtration over time.

According to the principles embraced in this book and in the work I do with clients, a kidney cleanse:

- Helps clear mineral buildup, sand, and retained deposits

- Supported filtration of both kidneys and related systems like ureters and pancreas

- Encourages improved fluid balance

- Reduces the workload on the immune system

- Supports overall detoxification pathways

When the kidneys begin to process more efficiently, the *entire system benefits* — from energy levels to circulation to immune response.

It's important to understand that kidney cleansing is **not something to be attempted casually or without guidance**. Just as with liver cleansing, a kidney cleanse should be **supervised, prepared, and individualized** so that the body can adapt safely. This helps reduce the risk of imbalance or discomfort during the process.

Hydration, Fluid Quality, and Balance

Hydration is essential for kidney function, but **more water is not always better**. In recent years, water consumption has been heavily promoted, often without enough attention to *quality, structure,* or *biological value.*

Today's water supply is largely depleted of natural minerals and frequently contaminated with chemicals, including fluoride and other residues. Standard refrigerator filters are not sufficient to remove many of these substances. For this reason, the *quality* of water matters just as much as the quantity.

Drinking large amounts of poorly structured, mineral-depleted water can place additional stress on the kidneys. Excess plain water may dilute the blood and contribute to the loss of important minerals and electrolytes, forcing the kidneys to work harder to maintain balance.

Clean, Structured Fluids Matter

For optimal kidney support, it is important to focus on **clean, living, and structured fluids**.

This includes:

- **Highly purified water**, properly filtered to remove chemicals such as fluoride

- **Structured water**, enhanced with natural elements that give it activity and mineral content

Simple ways to add structure and vitality to water include:

- A pinch of **Celtic sea salt**

- Fresh **lemon**

- A small amount of **raw apple cider vinegar**

These additions provide trace minerals, improve conductivity, and help water interact more effectively with the body rather than passing through as an empty fluid.

Biological Fluids Are Often Superior

From a biological standpoint, the body responds best to fluids that already contain nutrients and enzymes.

Freshly squeezed vegetable and fruit juices are examples of bioactive fluids that:

- Provide hydration

- Deliver minerals and electrolytes

- Support kidney filtration

- Reduce the need for excessive plain water intake

These fluids are recognized by the body as nourishment rather than dilution.

Hydration Is About Balance, Not Volume

Healthy hydration supports kidney function by providing the right fluids in the right form — not by overwhelming the system.

Rather than focusing on drinking large quantities of plain water, it is more supportive to:

- Prioritize fluid quality

- Include mineralized and structured liquids

- Use juices strategically

- Listen to the body's signals

When fluids are biologically active and mineral-rich, the kidneys can filter more efficiently with less strain. Watch the output. If your urine release is clear it means your blood has been heavily diluted and stripped. You are most likely drinking too much of poorly structured liquid.

What I Have Observed in Practice

In my work, I have seen that people often underestimate

how significantly the kidneys affect overall energy, fluid balance, and immune resilience. Many come in experiencing:

- Low energy

- Frequent urination patterns

- Back tension

- Swelling or fluid retention

- Frequent infections

- Mineral imbalance complaints

Once the kidneys receive appropriate support through hydration, dietary adjustments, and guided cleansing work, many clients report noticeable changes in energy, clarity, and a sense of internal lightness.

These improvements often emerge quietly — not dramatic or overwhelming, but steady and stabilizing.

Kidneys and the Body's Rhythms

Kidneys are closely tied to the body's fluid and metabolic cycles. Because they regulate electrolytes and waste removal, their function is sensitive to patterns of hydration, sleep, stress, and activity.

Supporting the kidneys with an appropriate fluid balance and avoiding chronic dehydration are foundational to long-term health and resilience.

Connecting the Kidneys to Other Systems

The kidneys do not operate in isolation. They are part of a network that includes:

- **The liver (filtration and chemical processing)**

- **The lymphatic system (fluid transport and defense)**

- **The digestive system (nutrient and waste balance)**

- **The cardiovascular system (blood pressure and flow)**

When kidney function improves, all of these systems feel some relief — because toxic load and fluid imbalance are reduced.

A Foundation for Later Chapters

As we continue, it will become clear that supporting organs like the kidneys is not an add-on or optional step — it is a

central pillar of whole-body balance. Effective cleansing and support in kidneys can facilitate deeper improvements in energy, detoxification, emotional regulation, and metabolic control.

Understanding the kidneys' role helps explain why the body can feel so different when filtration is supported correctly — not just for a moment, but over the long term.

SELF HELP KIDNEY MAINTENANCE:

Make juice: 12oz of carrot, 4 oz of beet, 4 oz of cucumber and 2 lemons. Mix the juice all together. Divide into 3 parts. Drink 3 times/day 20-30 minutes before meal for 7 days.

** For all kidney problems or disorders:*

• *Avoid salty and spicy foods.*

• *Eat watermelon as often as possible.*

• *Drink diuretic teas, such as rose hips, dandelion leaf, parsley.*

• Fresh watermelon juice (while in season).

Chapter 9: The Lymphatic System — Flow, Immunity, and Congestion

The lymphatic system is one of the most misunderstood systems in the body, yet it plays a central role in immunity, detoxification, and overall resilience.

Unlike the cardiovascular system, which has the heart to keep blood moving, the lymphatic system has no pump. It relies on movement, breathing, muscle contraction, and organ function to circulate lymph fluid throughout the body. When this flow slows or becomes congested, waste accumulates quietly — often long before symptoms appear.

The lymphatic system is not just about fighting infections. It is about **transport, clearance, and protection**.

What the Lymphatic System Does

The lymphatic system acts as the body's internal drainage network. It collects excess fluid, metabolic waste, toxins, cellular debris, and immune byproducts from tissues and returns them to the bloodstream for processing and elimination.

Lymph fluid passes through lymph nodes, where immune cells monitor, filter, and respond to potential threats. In this way, the lymphatic system connects detoxification and immunity into a single, continuous process.

When lymph flow is efficient, the body clears waste quietly and effectively. When it is sluggish, congestion builds.

Why Lymph Congestion Is So Common

Modern lifestyles are not friendly to lymphatic flow.

Long periods of sitting, shallow breathing, lack of movement, chronic stress, dehydration, and organ congestion all slow lymph circulation. Unlike blood, lymph does not circulate automatically. It must be moved.

When the liver, kidneys, or colon are overloaded, the lymphatic system often becomes a holding area for excess waste. Over time, this stagnation can contribute to swelling, tenderness, frequent infections, skin issues, and a general sense of heaviness in the body.

Many people experience lymph congestion without realizing it — because it does not always cause immediate pain.

The Lymphatic System and Immunity

The immune system depends heavily on lymphatic flow.

Immune cells travel through lymph fluid. Waste products from immune responses are also carried away through the lymphatic system. When lymph stagnates, immune responses may become inefficient or exaggerated.

This can show up as:

- Frequent colds or infections

- Allergic tendencies

- Chronic inflammation

- Slow recovery from illness

Supporting lymph flow is not about "boosting" immunity, but about allowing immune processes to function efficiently and clear waste once their job is done.

Fluid Balance and Lymph Flow

The lymphatic system works closely with the kidneys and circulatory system to manage fluid balance.

When fluids are poorly structured, mineral-depleted, or consumed in excess, lymph movement can slow. When kidneys are overloaded, lymph becomes an alternative storage route for waste that cannot be eliminated efficiently.

This is why supporting kidney filtration and choosing biologically active fluids helps lymph flow indirectly — by reducing the burden placed on the system.

Movement Is Medicine for the Lymph

Because the lymphatic system has no pump, **movement is essential**.

Walking, gentle stretching, deep breathing, and rhythmic activity stimulate lymph circulation. Even small amounts of regular movement can make a meaningful difference in how the body clears waste.

This is one reason people often feel lighter, clearer, and more energized after consistent movement — not because calories were burned, but because lymph finally moved.

What I Have Observed in Practice

In practice, I often see that when lymphatic congestion begins to clear, people notice changes that are subtle but significant.

Swelling decreases. Skin tone improves. The body feels less heavy. Recovery from illness becomes faster. Energy stabilizes.

These changes often occur alongside improvements in liver, kidney, and colon function, reinforcing the idea that the lymphatic system does not work alone — it responds to the overall internal environment.

Why Lymph Support Is Foundational

The lymphatic system connects all organs and tissues. When it is congested, no system is fully supported. When it flows, the body has a greater capacity to adapt, repair, and regulate itself.

Supporting lymph flow is not about aggressive intervention. It is about:

- Reducing overall toxic load

- Encouraging movement and circulation

- Supporting filtration organs

- Respecting the body's natural rhythms

When these conditions are met, the lymphatic system does what it was designed to do.

Preparing for Hormonal Balance

Hormones travel through blood and lymph. Waste hormones are also cleared through detox pathways that involve the liver, kidneys, and lymphatic system.

For this reason, hormonal balance cannot be fully addressed without first supporting filtration and flow.

The next chapter brings these systems together, exploring how the thyroid, adrenals, and sex hormones respond to stress, congestion, and detox capacity.

Lymph Cleansing Beverage.

Mix together:

4oz of beet juice

4oz of carrot juice

4oz of honey

4 oz of vodka

To consume:

Mix 2 table spoons of the solution in 4 oz of water and take 3 times/ day before meals, until the whole jar is gone.

Also see book Healing Through Cleansing 3 for daily Lymph cleansing techniques. Periodically, repeat herbal parasite cleansing to kill infection.

Super Blood Cleanser

Wash thoroughly and grind together in the blender or in the meat grinder:

12 oz of dried apricots

12 oz of black raisins

12 oz walnuts

12 oz honey

Mix well together and store in the refrigerator.

Take 1 tablespoon for 6 months in the morning on empty stomach.

Chapter 10: Hormones — Thyroid, Adrenals, and Sex Hormones

Hormones are messengers. They carry instructions from one part of the body to another, telling tissues when to activate, slow down, repair, reproduce, or rest. When hormones are balanced, the body feels coordinated and resilient. When they are not, the body feels confused, exhausted, and reactive.

Hormonal imbalance is rarely the result of a single gland malfunctioning. More often, it reflects a system under chronic strain.

Hormones Respond to the Internal Environment

Hormones do not operate independently. They respond to blood quality, liver filtration, lymphatic flow, digestive efficiency, stress levels, and toxin load.

When detox pathways are overwhelmed, hormones linger longer than intended. When filtration is sluggish, spent hormones are not cleared efficiently. When stress is constant, hormonal signaling shifts toward survival rather than balance.

This is why addressing hormones alone — without addressing the systems that regulate and clear them — often brings limited or temporary relief.

The Thyroid — Pace and Metabolism

The thyroid sets the metabolic pace of the body. It influences energy production, body temperature, weight regulation, digestion, mood, and mental clarity.

Thyroid function depends heavily on:

- Liver conversion of inactive hormones into active forms

- Adequate mineral availability

- Stable blood sugar

- Reduced inflammatory and toxic burden

When the liver is congested or the gut is inflamed, thyroid signaling may slow — even if laboratory values appear "normal."

In practice, many people with thyroid symptoms are not dealing with a thyroid problem alone, but with an environment that no longer supports proper thyroid expression.

The Adrenals — Stress and Survival

The adrenal glands respond to stress. They help regulate cortisol, adrenaline, and the body's ability to adapt to physical, emotional, and environmental challenges.

In a state of constant stress — whether from workload, emotional strain, poor sleep, or overstimulation — the adrenals remain active for too long. Over time, this disrupts hormonal balance throughout the body.

Chronic adrenal stress can affect:

- Blood sugar regulation

- Thyroid signaling

- Sex hormone production

- Immune resilience

- Sleep and recovery

The body prioritizes survival first. Balance comes later — if resources allow.

Sex Hormones — Cycles and Communication

Estrogen, progesterone, and testosterone influence reproduction, mood, bone health, libido, cognition, and tissue repair.

These hormones are meant to fluctuate rhythmically. Problems arise when they accumulate, dominate, or fail to clear.

The liver plays a critical role in breaking down and eliminating used sex hormones. When liver function is compromised, estrogen dominance and hormonal imbalance become more likely — in both women and men.

This imbalance may show up as:

- PMS or irregular cycles

- Menopausal symptoms

- Mood swings

- Weight changes

- Low libido

- Fatigue or irritability

These symptoms are not isolated failures. They are signals of a system under strain.

Hormones and Detoxification

Hormones are not only produced — they must also be **cleared**. Spent hormones are processed by the liver, transported through lymph, and eliminated through the kidneys and colon. When any part of this pathway is congested, hormones remain active longer than intended.

This is why detoxification capacity plays such a critical role in hormonal balance.

Women with hot flashes improve their symptoms greatly or eliminate them completely with each liver cleanse and following mainly a vegetarian diet. Eating meat plays a big role in producing access heat and iron that the body is trying to push out through the sweat.

Men with erectile disfunction and or low testosterone levels see quick results after detoxing their liver and following dietary recommendations.

In practice, I often observe that hormonal symptoms improve only after detox pathways are supported — not because hormones are being forced into balance, but because the body regains its ability to regulate naturally.

Stress, Media, and Hormonal Noise

Modern stress is not only physical. Continuous mental stimulation, media exposure, emotional overload, and constant decision-making all influence hormonal signaling.

The nervous system communicates directly with hormonal glands. When the nervous system never fully settles, hormones remain in a state of response rather than regulation.

This creates a background "noise" that interferes with hormonal rhythm and recovery.

What I Have Observed in Practice

Many people seek help for hormonal imbalance believing it to be a glandular issue. Over time, it becomes clear that when digestion improves, detoxification pathways open, lymph flow increases, and stress load decreases, hormones often begin to stabilize on their own.

This does not happen overnight. It happens gradually — as pressure is removed from the system.

Hormones respond best to **support**, not force.

Hormones as Messengers, Not Enemies

Hormonal symptoms are often viewed as problems to suppress. In reality, they are messages indicating that the internal environment has changed.

Listening to these messages allows for a more intelligent approach — one that restores balance by addressing root causes rather than chasing numbers.

Preparing for Nourishment

Hormones are built from nutrients. The quality, timing, and composition of food directly influence hormonal expression, detoxification, and recovery.

The next chapter explores food and nutrition — not as rigid rules, but as daily support for every system discussed so far.

Chapter 11: The Nervous System

Stress, Safety, and the Body's Ability to Heal

The nervous system is the master regulator of the body. It determines how we digest, how we detoxify, how we repair, and how we respond to the world around us. No organ functions independently of it. When the nervous system is balanced, the body adapts with resilience. When it is overstimulated or locked in survival mode, healing slows — even when everything else appears to be in place.

This is why two people can follow the same diet, take the same supplements, or undergo similar therapies and experience very different outcomes. The difference often lies not in what they are doing, but in the state of their nervous system.

Two States: Survival and Restoration

The nervous system operates primarily through two opposing states.

One state is designed for **action, alertness, and protection**. It prepares the body to respond quickly, increasing heart rate, tightening muscles, diverting blood away from digestion, and heightening awareness. This response is necessary and life-saving in moments of danger.

The other state is responsible for **restoration, digestion, detoxification, and repair**. In this state, blood flow returns to the digestive organs, hormones regulate more smoothly, immune function stabilizes, and tissues regenerate.

The body is meant to move fluidly between these states. Problems arise when the nervous system remains chronically locked in the first.

Why the Nervous System Becomes Overloaded

Unlike physical threats, modern stressors are often constant and unresolved. The body does not distinguish between emotional pressure, mental overload, or physical danger — it simply responds.

Continuous stimulation, information exposure, emotional processing without release, and lack of true rest keep the nervous system activated. Over time, this activation becomes the body's default setting.

When this happens:

- Digestion becomes weaker

- Detoxification slows

- Immune responses become exaggerated or
  suppressed

- Hormonal rhythms lose precision

- Inflammation becomes chronic

The body is not malfunctioning — it is prioritizing survival over repair.

The Nervous System and Digestion

Digestion is one of the first functions to be compromised under stress. The stomach, small intestine, pancreas, liver, and colon all rely on parasympathetic nervous system activity to function properly.

When the nervous system senses threat or pressure:

- Stomach acid production drops or becomes
  imbalanced

- Enzyme secretion weakens

- Peristalsis slows or becomes irregular

- Nutrient absorption is reduced

This creates a cascade effect. Food is not properly broken down, residues remain in the digestive tract, and toxins recirculate rather than being eliminated. Over time, this contributes to congestion in the gut, liver overload, microbial imbalance, and systemic inflammation.

Emotional Processing and the Body

The nervous system is also the interface between emotional experience and physical response. Emotions are not stored in the brain as abstract concepts — they are experienced and recorded through the body.

When emotions are processed and released, the nervous system resets. When they are suppressed, rushed, or continuously stimulated without resolution, the body holds tension.

This tension does not remain theoretical. It alters muscle tone, organ function, circulation, and energy flow. Over time, emotional strain becomes physical strain — not because emotions are harmful, but because unresolved activation keeps the body from returning to a restorative state.

Why Healing Can Stall

Many people do "everything right" and still struggle to heal. They eat well, avoid obvious toxins, and follow structured protocols — yet progress remains limited.

In these cases, the nervous system may not perceive safety. Without safety, the body will not prioritize detoxification, regeneration, or deep repair.

This is not a conscious decision. It is biological intelligence.

The body will always choose protection before purification.

Observations from Practice

In working with clients, I have observed that when the nervous system begins to settle, other systems respond almost immediately. Digestion improves. Sleep deepens. Emotional resilience increases. Detoxification becomes more efficient — not because force is applied, but because resistance is removed.

This is also why some individuals experience emotional release during physical cleansing or bodywork. When the nervous system shifts from holding to releasing, the body lets go of more than just physical waste.

These responses are not random. They are signs of regulation returning.

Supporting the Nervous System

Supporting the nervous system does not require constant effort or drastic change. Often, it involves removing excess stimulation and allowing the body to complete cycles it has been holding open.

Simple, consistent signals of safety — warmth, rhythm, regular nourishment, rest, and presence — allow the nervous system to shift naturally.

When this happens, the body does what it was designed to do.

The Foundation of All Healing

Every system discussed in this book — digestive, detoxification, hormonal, immune — depends on the nervous system's ability to regulate.

Without nervous system support, healing becomes an uphill effort. With it, the body regains access to its inherent intelligence.

This is not about controlling the body. It is about allowing it.

Moving Forward

With an understanding of how regulation influences every organ system, we are now ready to bring everything together through **Food and Nutrition** — not as rules or trends, but as daily signals that support digestion, detoxification, and balance at the most fundamental level.

Chapter 12: Diet and Nutrition — Simplicity, Purity, and Intelligent Nourishment

True healing nutrition is not complicated. It is disciplined simplicity.

The human body is not designed to interpret dozens of ingredients at once. Each food carries its own chemical, enzymatic, and energetic signature. When too many different foods are introduced simultaneously, even if they are individually healthy, the digestive system becomes confused, efficiency drops, and the organs of filtration and elimination are forced to compensate.

This is why complex meals so often lead to fatigue, heaviness, bloating, and long-term metabolic strain.

The Body Thrives on Clarity

Simple meals allow the stomach to secrete the appropriate acids, the pancreas to release the correct enzymes, and the intestines to absorb nutrients effectively. Complexity creates competition. Simplicity creates nourishment.

Ingredient Integrity

The body recognizes food — not chemistry.

Anything artificial that enters the body must be neutralized, transformed, or removed. Artificial colors, flavors, preservatives, pesticides, solvents, medications, smoke, alcohol, and environmental fumes all pass through the bloodstream and must be filtered, primarily by the liver.

The liver's task is not only to process nutrients but to protect the blood from substances that do not belong in it. Over time, these substances accumulate and begin to clog the body's natural filters.

This is why ingredient quality is not optional.

Organic foods reduce the chemical load placed on the liver, gallbladder, kidneys, and lymphatic system. Genetically modified foods further complicate this burden, as they often contain residues and altered proteins that the immune and detoxification systems struggle to recognize and process.

Whenever possible, choose foods that are:

• Organic

• Whole

- Minimally processed

- Fresh

- Free of chemical additives

This is not a lifestyle trend. It is a physiological necessity for detoxification and regeneration.

Living vs. Dead Nutrition

Living foods carry life force.

Fresh vegetables, fruits, greens, sprouts, and whole plant foods contain enzymes, structured water, antioxidants, and micronutrients that actively participate in cellular repair.

Dead foods — refined, preserved, chemically altered, and excessively cooked — may provide calories, but they no longer provide biological intelligence. They burden the digestive system, slow elimination, and contribute to stagnation within the tissues. Same happens from the microwave use. Besides radiation and harmful EMFs, micro-waves heat the food without heat by spinning the molecules so fast that the substance heats up itself. That action completely and irreversibly changes the structure of water or product heated. So even an organic healthy food once heated in the microwave becomes dead, has zero nutritional value, genetically modified and unrecognizable by your body.

Healing occurs when the majority of the diet is composed of living foods.

A primarily plant-based diet is not a moral position. It is a biological one.

Animal protein is dense, slow to digest, and highly demanding on the liver and kidneys. For most people, frequent consumption prevents cleansing and regeneration. When used, it should be limited, intentional, and infrequent — ideally no more than once or twice weekly, and often less during healing phases.

Are Humans Meant to Eat Meat?

This question is often framed emotionally or ideologically. A more useful approach is to examine human biology calmly and honestly.

From a biological perspective, humans are omnivores with a strong plant bias. We are not obligate carnivores, nor are we strict herbivores. We fall somewhere in between — but much closer to plant-eaters than to predators in anatomy, digestion, and physiology.

This distinction matters.

Carnivorous animals are designed to hunt and tear flesh. They possess long, sharp canines, blade-like teeth for slicing meat, minimal grinding surfaces, and jaws that move primarily up and down. Their digestive tracts are short, and their stomach acid is extremely acidic to prevent putrefaction of dense animal tissue.

Herbivores, in contrast, have small or absent canines, broad flat molars for grinding plants, and jaws capable of side-to-side and circular motion. Their digestive systems are long and designed for fermentation and gradual breakdown of plant material.

Humans clearly do not fit the carnivore model. Our canines are small and blunt, not fangs. We have large flat molars for grinding. Our jaws move side-to-side and forward and back. Tooth wear patterns in humans resemble those of fruit- and plant-eating primates far more than predators.

Digestive anatomy reinforces this. Human intestines are approximately ten to twelve times body length — far longer than carnivores — and stomach acidity is moderate rather than extreme. This means food remains in the system longer. Under these conditions, plant foods ferment beneficially, while heavy animal foods tend to stagnate and putrefy when consumed frequently or in excess.

Human biochemistry tells the same story. We produce salivary amylase to begin digesting starches in the mouth — an enzyme carnivores largely lack. We do not efficiently produce enzymes to break down raw animal fat or collagen. Our enzyme profile favors roots, fruits, greens, and starches.

Vitamin arguments are often misunderstood. Vitamin B12, for example, does not originate in animals but in soil bacteria. Animals accumulate it by consuming soil-contaminated plants. Humans historically obtained B12 the same way, but modern sanitation removed this source. This represents an environmental mismatch, not proof that humans are biologically designed to consume meat.

From an evolutionary perspective, early humans ate predominantly plants, fruits, tubers, and seeds. Animal foods were eaten opportunistically — insects, eggs, scavenged meat — not as a dietary foundation. The use of tools and fire expanded what humans could eat, but cooking changed capability, not biological design.

Population-level data aligns with this anatomy. Diets rich in whole plant foods consistently correlate with lower rates of chronic disease. Diets high in animal protein and fat correlate with increased cardiovascular disease, diabetes, colon cancer, kidney strain, and inflammatory conditions.

The conclusion is this:

Humans are adaptive *omnivores by survival,* but primarily *plant-eaters by biology.*

We can eat meat, but we are not optimized for heavy or frequent meat consumption.

We thrive best when plant foods dominate, with animal foods remaining optional, occasional, or culturally driven.

Biology is not about what is possible. It is about what supports optimal function over time.

The Protein Myth

The fear of protein deficiency is largely cultural, not physiological.

Every plant contains amino acids. Many plant foods, particularly leafy greens, legumes, quinoa, and buckwheat, provide protein in a form that is already biologically available.

Unlike animal protein, which must be broken down into amino acids before use, plant protein is assimilated with minimal digestive effort. This conserves metabolic energy and reduces toxic byproducts.

True strength is not built from overload — it is built from efficient nourishment.

Juicing as Cellular Medicine

Juicing is not a trend.

It is therapeutic nutrition.

Fresh juices deliver minerals, vitamins, enzymes, and phytochemicals directly to the bloodstream through the stomach lining. This bypasses many digestive inefficiencies caused by inflammation, enzyme depletion, malabsorption, and intestinal imbalance.

For this reason, juices must be consumed on an empty stomach.

Juice is not digested. It is absorbed.

This is why it is such a powerful tool in cleansing, rebuilding, and disease reversal.

Vegetable-based juices are the foundation. Fruit may be used strategically, not excessively.

Certain juices demonstrate consistent therapeutic value:

Carrot juice exhibits strong anti-parasitic, anti-fungal, and growth-inhibiting properties and has been extensively used in supportive cancer care.

Carrot and celery juice dissolves mucus and is especially beneficial in respiratory and inflammatory conditions.

Carrot, beet, and green apple juice supports liver regeneration, bile flow, and the gradual dissolution of hepatic and gallbladder congestion when used consistently and correctly.

Green juices provide readily available amino acids and cleanse the blood at a cellular level.

Juicing, when practiced with structure and intention, nourishes and cleanses simultaneously.

Smoothies — Nutritional Density, Not Same as Juice

Smoothies are blended food. They require digestion.

Their value lies in their ability to deliver large quantities of greens and plant matter that might otherwise be difficult to consume. Their limitation lies in the absence of chewing and salivary enzyme activation.

Smoothies support nutrition. They do not replace cleansing.

They should be used as meals, not as medicinal tools.

Intelligent Hydration

The day should begin with a glass of water — always at room or body temperature, never cold.

Ideally, add the juice of half a lemon or one teaspoon of apple cider vinegar. A small pinch of Celtic salt is also an excellent addition.

Modern water is highly processed. Filtration removes harmful substances, but it also strips water of its natural minerals and vitality. What remains is often "dead" water — clean, but empty.

This is why electrolyte waters have become such a large industry. Yet true remineralization does not require expensive products. A pinch of high-quality salt, such as Celtic salt, added to your water is often sufficient to restore mineral content and improve hydration at the cellular level.

Drinking large quantities of plain, demineralized water does not necessarily hydrate the body. In fact, excessive "empty" water can dilute the blood and strip essential minerals from tissues. I regularly see individuals who consume a gallon of water daily yet continue to exhibit clear signs of dehydration.

More is not always better. Even water, in excess, becomes harmful. There are well-documented cases where extreme fluid intake has led to serious electrolyte imbalance and, in rare situations, fatal outcomes. Moderation is essential in every aspect of health.

A simple and affordable method of mineral support is to place a few grains of Celtic salt directly in the mouth, allow them to dissolve, and follow with a few sips of water. This delivers minerals in a highly bioavailable form

Hydration must support digestion, not sabotage it

Drinking large amounts of liquid during meals dilutes gastric acid and enzymes, cools the digestive environment, and forces the stomach to empty prematurely.

This creates fermentation, bloating, and nutrient loss.

Cold beverages are particularly disruptive, as the body must divert energy to rewarm the stomach before digestion can occur.

The most supportive practice is pre-meal hydration.

A warm or room-temperature drink 20–30 minutes before eating prepares the stomach, stimulates secretions, and reduces overeating.

Small sips of warm tea may be tolerated with meals. Large volumes should not.

If you are intensely thirsty during or immediately after eating, the food is not serving you.

Overeating and Metabolic Congestion

When the stomach is overloaded, digestion stops.

Undigested material is passed into the intestines, which are not designed to process it. This disrupts absorption, burdens elimination, and contributes to systemic toxicity.

Healing requires space — not excess.

The Therapeutic Value of the Evening Fast

Nighttime is the body's primary repair cycle.

Late or heavy meals interrupt this process. The liver remains in digestive mode instead of detoxification and regeneration.

For optimal healing:

- Eat early

- Eat lightly

- Eat plant-based in the evening

• Or consider eliminating dinner during therapeutic phases

Animal protein is best consumed at midday, when digestive strength is highest.

Food Combining and Fruit Physiology

Fruit is designed to move quickly.

When eaten alone, it digests efficiently and nourishes the body. When eaten with other foods, it becomes trapped, ferments, feeds pathogenic organisms, and produces gas and discomfort.

Fruit should be eaten on an empty stomach.

Melons are even more rapid in digestion.

All melons may be combined with each other — except watermelon, which should be eaten completely alone.

Watermelon is a powerful kidney cleanser, hydrator, and mineral source. When used correctly, it supports elimination and renal function. When used incorrectly, it ferments and becomes destabilizing.

Follow the physiology, and fruit becomes medicine.

The Rhythm of Eating

The body does not function randomly. It moves in cycles of activity, digestion, cleansing, and repair. When eating becomes constant, irregular, or emotionally driven, these natural rhythms are disrupted.

Frequent snacking does not support healing. It keeps the digestive system in continuous work and prevents the organs from completing their restorative functions.

Regular, intentional meals allow the stomach, liver, pancreas, and intestines to work efficiently and then rest. This rhythm builds strength rather than exhaustion.

Hunger should be respected. Appetite driven by stress, fatigue, or habit should be observed. The body heals in the spaces between meals as much as it does during nourishment.

Inflammation or Nourishment

Every food creates a response.

Some foods calm tissues, support circulation, and reduce irritation. Others inflame, congest, and burden the system.

Inflammation is not always dramatic. It often feels like heaviness, fog, stiffness, swelling, discomfort, and fatigue.

A healing diet is not defined only by nutrients, but by how the body feels after eating.

When food consistently leaves the body clearer, lighter, and more stable, healing is taking place.

Mineral Balance and Internal Acidity

Modern diets are mineral-poor and chemically demanding.

Processed foods, sugar, excessive animal protein, and refined products increase metabolic acidity. To neutralize this, the body draws minerals from its own reserves — bones, tissues, and organs.

Mineral-rich plant foods, especially greens, vegetables, and fresh juices, buffer this acidity and support cellular function.

Healing nutrition replenishes minerals before stimulating the body.

Food as Information

Food is not only fuel. It is biological instruction.

Every meal communicates with hormones, immune cells, the nervous system, and metabolism. It programs inflammatory responses, blood sugar regulation, energy production, and emotional stability.

What we eat becomes how the body thinks, reacts, and heals.

This is why diet is never neutral.

Healing Nutrition vs. Maintenance Nutrition

There is a difference between eating to maintain and eating to heal.

During periods of fatigue, illness, hormonal imbalance, detoxification, or emotional strain, the body requires lighter, simpler, more digestible nourishment.

Liquid nutrition, plant-based meals, and reduced protein load allow energy to be redirected from digestion to repair.

As strength returns, the diet can broaden — but healing must come first.

Sensitivity and Body Intelligence

The body constantly communicates.

Bloating, fatigue, cravings, mood changes, skin reactions, and energy shifts after eating are not random. They are feedback.

Learning to observe these responses builds internal awareness and guides intelligent choice.

No universal diet can replace personal physiological understanding.

Consistency Over Perfection

Healing does not require perfection.

It requires direction, repetition, and patience.

Occasional deviation does not undo progress. Chronic disregard does.

Small, consistent choices create deep change.

The body responds to what is done most often, not what is done occasionally.

Healthy Recipes Examples

Homemade Granola

Ingredients

- 3 ½ Cups Old Fashioned Rolled Oats (Gluten-Free if Needed)

- 1 Cup Almonds

- 1 Cup Pecans

- 1 Cup Pistachios

- ½ Cup Raw Pumpkin Seeds

- ½ Cup Raw Sunflower Seeds

- 2 Tsp Pumpkin Pie Spice

- 1 ½ Tsp Sea Salt

- ⅔ Cup Pure Maple Syrup

- 1/2 cup coconut oil melted

- 1 ½ Cups Golden Raisins

- 1 ½ Cups Dried Cranberries

Step 1: Preheat Your Oven

Begin by preheating your oven to 325 degrees.

Step 2: Combine Dry Ingredients.

In a large bowl, mix oats, nuts, seeds, pumpkin pie spice, and salt. Set aside.

Step 3: Mix Syrup

Mix maple syrup and coconut oil together.

Step 4: pour over the dry ingredients, mix well, put on the lined baking sheet, press down

Bake for 16 minutes, stir, then bake another 10 minutes. Add the raisins and cranberries, and return to the oven for another 10 minutes.

Mango Overnight Oats

Ingredients

- ½ cup Rolled Oats

- 1 tablespoon Maple Syrup (optional for sweetening)

- 1 teaspoon Chia Seeds

- ½ teaspoon Lime Juice (or more to taste)

- ¼ teaspoon Ground Cardamom or Cinnamon

- Pinch of Salt

- ½ cup coconut milk (or your favorite plant-based milk)

- ¼ cup Diced Mango (fresh, canned in water, or frozen and thawed will work)

- ¼ cup Unsweetened Coconut Yogurt (or your favorite plant-based yogurt)

Optional Toppings

- Optional toppings:

- Diced Mango or any other fruit of your choice

- Sliced Almonds or other nuts of your choice

- Toasted Coconut

Instructions

Mix the Base

In a jar or small bowl (at least 10 ounces), add rolled oats, maple syrup (if using), chia seeds, lime juice, cardamom, salt, and coconut milk. Stir well to make sure everything is evenly distributed.

Add Mango

Gently fold in the diced mango. Don't mash it. You want those juicy chunks intact.

Add Yogurt

Spoon the coconut yogurt on top without stirring it in just yet. This helps keep the layers distinct and makes for a prettier presentation if you're prepping ahead.

Refrigerate

Cover and refrigerate for at least 2 hours, but ideally overnight (8– 12 hours). This is when the magic happens. The oats absorb the liquid, the flavors mingle, and everything transforms into creamy perfection.

Serve

When you're ready to eat, stir in the yogurt to create extra creaminess. Add your favorite toppings, and enjoy straight from the jar or in a bowl.

Greek Chickpea Quinoa Salad

This Greek Chickpea and Quinoa Salad is a vibrant, protein-packed dish with fresh veggies, perfect for meal prep, potlucks, or a quick, healthy meal.

Ingredients

- *1 cup uncooked quinoa*

- *1 15 ounce can of chickpeas, drained and rinsed*

- *1 cup cucumbers, chopped*

- *1 cup cherry tomatoes, sliced*

- *¼ cup red onion, diced*

- *1 red or yellow bell pepper, diced*

- *Artichoke Hearts (optional)*

- *pepperoncini's (optional)*

- *olives (optional)*

- *Olive, Flex or Sesame oil, lemon and or Bragg Aminos (soy sauce alternative).*

Instructions

1. *Bring 2 cups of water to a boil.*

2. *Rinse quinoa in a fine mesh strainer before adding to water.*

3. *Cook quinoa according to the package directions, feel free to add veggie broth mix to your water if you want more flavor.*

4. *While the quinoa is cooking, chop your veggies, drain the chickpeas and make your salad dressing.*

5. *Once quinoa is cooked, mix in the veggies, chickpeas and salad dressing. Stir well.*

6. *Store in the refrigerator for a few days.*

Hearty Veggie Soup

This Hearty Veggie Soup is an easy plant-based recipe your family will love. Beans, potatoes and broccoli plus more veggie goodness.

Ingredients

- 1 cup diced onion

- 2 cloves garlic, minced

- 3 carrots, sliced

- 3 stalks celery, sliced

- 4 peeled and diced potatoes (about 5-6 cups)

- 1 cup frozen green beans

- 1 crown broccoli, chopped (about 2-3 cups)

- 1 15 oz can black beans, drained and rinsed

- 1 15 oz can petite diced tomatoes

- 8 cups of water or broth (if using water, add veggie broth mix)

- Salt and pepper to taste

Instructions

1. Begin to saute the onions and garlic. Add a little water if needed. This makes the house smell glorious!

2. Add the carrots and celery. Then dump in the potatoes, green beans, and broccoli.

3. *Cover the veggie with water or veggie broth, I use about 8 cups of water and add 8-10 tablespoons of my Veggie Broth Mix.*

4. *Pour in the diced tomatoes and black beans.*

5. *Cover with a lid and simmer for 30-45 minutes, until all the veggies are soft.*

6. *Salt and pepper if desired.*

Triple Berry Frozen Yogurt Pops

Ingredients

- *½ cup regular or non-dairy yogurt*

- *1 cup of fresh berries*

- *sweetener (optional)*

Instructions

1. *Pour ½ cup of non-dairy yogurt into a blender.*

2. *Pour in half of the berries.*

3. *Blend in blender until smooth.*

4. *Taste and add sweetener if needed. I recommend maple syrup or stevia then blend again.*

5. *Once appropriately sweet, spoon into freezer molds until ¾ of the way full.*

6. *Carefully drop berries into the molds using whole blueberries, diced strawberries and halved blackberries.*

7. *Place sticks into the molds and freeze over night.*

8. *To loosen freezer pops, dip the molds into warm water then gently pull out the freezer pops.*

9. *Store in the freezer until ready to eat.*

Tomato Soup

Ingredients

- *Extra-virgin olive oil*

- *2 pint (about 650 grams) cherry tomatoes*

- *1 yellow onion, roughly chopped*

- *1 small garlic head, halved crosswise*

- *1 bunch basil*

- *1 bunch thyme*

- *1 red chile, optional*

- *Salt and pepper*

- *1/2 cup full-fat coconut milk, soy cream, or heavy cream*

- *1/2 cup vegetable stock, plus more as needed*

Directions

- *Heat the oven to 480°F (250°C).*

- *Drizzle some oil into a deep baking dish. Add in the onion, garlic (cut side down), basil and thyme, chile, and tomatoes. Drizzle more olive oil on top, plus a big sprinkle of salt and pepper. Bake for 25 to 35 minutes, until the tomatoes are slightly charred.*

- *Let cool for 5 to 7 minutes. Remove and discard the thyme. Add the rest of the ingredients to a blender, along with the coconut milk and vegetable stock. Remove the little plug from the blender lid, then cover the lid with a kitchen towel and blend until smooth. Taste and adjust the salt and pepper if needed.*

- *Serve with a piece of buttered toast or a grilled cheese sandwich.*

CONCLUSION

Listening Forward

Healing is not a destination.

It is a relationship.

A relationship with the body, with rhythm, with nourishment, with rest, and with awareness.

Throughout this book, we have explored how the digestive system reflects the larger story of modern life — overload, imbalance, compensation, and resilience. What becomes clear is this:

The body is not broken.

It is responding. Symptoms are not failures. They are intelligent adaptations.

When we stop fighting the body and begin supporting it, something profound happens. The system begins to reorganize. Energy returns. Clarity improves. Inflammation settles. The body remembers how to heal.

True healing does not come from force, restriction, or fear.

It comes from simplicity, consistency, and respect for the body's natural design.

For those who feel they need deeper, structured support, professional guidance can be invaluable. Comprehensive cleansing and restoration programs, when done correctly, address not one organ but the entire internal environment — digestion, detoxification, elimination, and immune balance together.

Healing is not about fixing parts. It is about restoring the whole.

If this book leaves you with one understanding, let it be this:

Your body is always working for you.

Your task is not to control it — but to understand it.

ABOUT THE AUTHOR

Dr. Elena Rybak, PhD, is a holistic health practitioner and educator specializing in digestive health, nutritional therapy, and internal detoxification.

Her work centers on the most comprehensive cleansing and restoration approaches available today — addressing the body as an integrated system rather than isolated symptoms. Through years of clinical practice, she has developed structured programs that support the liver, intestines, lymphatic system, and metabolic balance in a coordinated and gentle way.

Elena offers individualized cleansing and healing programs that can be completed from anywhere in the United States, allowing clients to receive guided support regardless of location.

More information about her work, educational resources, and available cleansing programs can be found at:

www.livinghealthyinstitute.com

Her philosophy is grounded in the belief that the body is intelligent, adaptive, and capable of deep repair when given the proper conditions.